A hole in the ear

Preface-

The purpose of this story is to describe what happens when a hole is found in the ear. This book will discuss the pain, the daily struggles, the hope, and the defeat. Somewhere in the book, the reader will find tips for the loved ones who live with this daily. It is not just a struggle for the person with the hole, it is a family struggle. This book will talk about the struggles I faced growing as a person and how in many ways the growth has just started. As I write this book I hope to find peace for myself, strength to push on and maybe help someone else who one September day was told they have a hole in their ear.

Chapter one-

Where it all began

This story begins just over a year ago, September 2017. I had been told a few times over recent months that I was talking loud. Wondering what it could be caused by, since I could not hear myself talking loud I made an appointment with Costco Hearing Center. Yes of all places, because it was free. I can remember thinking the week before the appointment, oh I am sure it is nothing. I will arrive they will test my hearing and just tell me I talk too loud.

Simple fix right just train yourself to talk quieter. Looking back now I wish that would have been the case more than anything. Instead, the first comment out of her mouth was "oh wow". After her statement, she proceeded to show me the image on her computer monitor of what she was seeing. I was shocked, to say the least, I clearly had a hole in my eardrum. With this knowledge, she suggested holding off on the hearing test and making an appointment with the ENT doctor as soon as possible. I remember thinking at the time how does that even happen. I was hoping that once I saw the ENT that she would say it is an easy fix, and you have no worries. Prior to my appointment that I had to wait several weeks for I spent a lot of time researching the internet ...by the way, this is a bad idea. Dr. Google only increases the worry. All it does is fuel the anxiety and really what can you believe off the internet.

Chapter 2

What happens next

After what seemed like an eternity I was able to make it to the ENT doctor. I can still remember the first thing she said: "wow that is a pretty good size hole, not the biggest one I have seen but close". She then sat down and talked with me about potential things that could have caused it. The doctor stated that several things that can cause a hole in your eardrum can range from long-term ear infections, loud explosions, injury, and eustachian tube dysfunction. It's a tough thing to analyze as it is not always crystal clear what is going on. At the time it was not clear to the Doctor what could have been the cause.

Our conversation continued to go along the path of what one should do next. For this size whole, there was no way that it would close on its own. It would likely only get larger if it was left alone. Really the only option was to perform surgery. During this visit, we discussed the risks, complications, success rate, and the doctor's overall opinion. She said it was a 90% chance the hole would restore some of the hearing that was lost. It was at this same visit that I was told I have a moderate hearing loss in my left ear which has the hole and mild hearing loss in my right ear. It was at this visit I found out why I was talking loud. While many might say, well at least you know. All I wanted to do after this appointment was cry. Which I allowed myself to do once I got in the car.

I decided at that appointment to think about having the surgery. The name of the surgery for those that like to research the internet was tympanoplasty. I had mostly decided I was going to do it, but had to give myself a day or so to really think about what that meant. What if something went wrong, or was it really worth the cost of the surgery. Knowing that it was a 90% chance that it would work had me leaning towards having it. After discussing it with a few trusted people in my life I decided this risk was worth the reward, or so I thought. Making the decision here is hard as there are many unknowns.

Chapter 3

Surgery Day

Surgery day I was brought to the surgery center by my boyfriend. I remember being scared, I have never liked being put to sleep. The anastigilogost came in and discussed with me my breathing and asthma history. At that time I become even more nervous as he said was going to place a breathing tube down my throat. He seemed to think was the best idea. All I could think about in that moment is was I wanted to run out the door. I have never liked being in hospitals or surgery centers. The surgery itself was explained that first they would cut behind the back of my ear and would take a patch of my skin and transplant it over my eardrum. They would then stitch my ear closed and put a plug over the patch inside the ear to hold it in place. I would wear something awkward and dorky over my ear for 4-5 days. I still can't believe I signed the consent forms and the surgery was performed.

Recovery

     I do not remember coming home that day. My boyfriend brought me home and sometime later that day I woke up with a pain in my ear and my throat. The pain quite possibly is the worst pain I have ever had. I literally thought wow I am feeling really low. Over the course of the next week, I spent a lot of time sleeping, waking and sleeping again. I was in pain, could not hear at all and basically felt worthless. I actually can't remember a time I felt this horrific. It was on the fifth day that I met my worst bought of nausea. I must have got sick like 10 times in the course of a very short period of time. Causing the need to go to the ER. I remember making a call to the on-call doctor since was a Saturday and the on-call doctor did nothing but make me feel anxious.

     The ER visit consisted of the doctor taking blood work and x-ray to make sure I was not having an infection or other issue related to the surgery, and a shot of morphine that made me want to die. I think I may have even stopped breathing for a second. Note to self always asks what they're giving you when they try putting something in an IV. If it is morphine take a hard pass. After the morphine, I passed out. Sometime after waking up I was given a nauseous patch which worked wonders in fixing nausea. I was then able to leave the emergency room and come home.

I remember the first day I left the house after that was to go out to dinner with boyfriend. I recall still being out of sorts, being in pain and feeling like I was actually pushing myself to go out as I had been in the house for an entire week pretty much just sleeping. As hard as it is, if you go through this surgery or another find some motivation to get out for a brief period and if you can't find the motivation hopefully someone in your life can help you as it I think it was important in the road to recovery.

The next several weeks were difficult in maintaining mental strength. Having the plug inside my ear, not being able to hear and having pain both inside and outside of the year pushed me hard. I can recall tears, pain, and just wanting to be silent because if I asked a question or tried to have a conversation hearing was beyond hard. Understanding that there would be a light at the end of the tunnel kept me centered. I recall looking many times over the course of not just those first few weeks but the last two years to a card that was given to me that encouraged me to be strong. I mean, at some point, the hearing would get better. That was my hope.

Chapter 4

Post recovery

All winter long there was a pain in the ear. The pain inside and pain at the incision site. I had to wear a beanie hat everywhere that I went. I felt awkward and sad. I wondered why me so many times during this process. I look back now and realize I think this is normal. Feeling pain mentally and physically and being sad is normal when someone is going through something like this. I know some people do not see this as a big deal. To those people, I say it is and if you have someone going through this or any health problem let it be that person who decides if it is a big deal or not.

After a month I was seen by the ENT to consider removing the plug in the ear, however, the doctor did not think it was ready. She wanted it left in a few more weeks. By this time it had gotten easier to have the plugin but was still annoying and I wanted it out. After the plug was finally removed there was still packing in the ear that would construct the hearing. I could still feel like I had something in my ear, but it was at least less foreign objects in my ear. Due to the packing being left, I had to wait to have hearing checked for another month. I was anxious to find out if there was some improvement, hopeful that my hearing would be better. That I would not talk loud at times where it was not appropriate.

When I had my hearing checked it was a defeating moment, not only had there been no improvement, my hearing had worsened. This was something that I already knew based on my daily activities, but I was hoping the data would show something different. It was at this point the doctor said there is a chance the improvement will not come, a hearing aid needed was a real possibility. This visit was where I knew life would be different and I had no control over it happening. I only had control of how I let it affect me, which at the time and even now as I write this is a struggle.

Over the months that followed I spent time listening, hoping that one moment would come where I would see improvement. Where I would wake up and hear better I spent time worrying in my mind, but not saying things out loud. Complaining did not seem to be a good answer. Instead I tried to have hope to believe. Sometimes however we do not get the answer we want. More shattering news was to come.

Chapter 5

Slx month later

I was preparing for a trip for work where I was flying into Nevada. A trip that all Branch managers attend annually, this was to be my one and likely only trip. I can remember being nervous to fly, more than my normal nervous. I was concerned that my ear was not ready for the trip and sought counsel from my ENT Doctor to determine if my ear was stable and could handle the flight. The concern was the change in altitude and the pressure building in my ear. I can remember specifically asking if this was your daughter flying would you give her the green light? As in how sure are you that my patch on the eardrum is completely healed...she gave the green light and off I went. I can remember wondering if I

was going to have blood spewing out of my ear in mid flight.
I did not bleed, but I had pain, I felt pressured. I kept telling
myself the doctor said this would be fine, but in the back of
my mind I was thinking I don't recall having ear pain this bad
in my previous flights.

In lieu of giving the details of the trip, I will skip to
several months after the trip. I had been having ear pain off
and on for a while so I decided to make an appointment
earlier than our pre-discussed appointment. This
appointment was shattering as it was where I found that a
section of the patch that was placed during my
tympanoplasty surgery had deteriorated. The surgery that is
supposed to be 90% successful had failed. The doctor's
theory is that my eustachian tubes cause pressure on the
eardrum and even if I had the surgery again it would likely
have a similar problem. I can remember this day well, I recall
leaving this appointment and sitting in the car first staring off
into space, and they just letting the tears fall. It pained me to

not know what to do, to feel like I had been given a raw deal. Not only did I have to worry about not regaining my hearing, but that they would likely get worse.

This is a moment that I will say being your own advocate is important. Looking back I wonder if I should not have been at such extreme elevations yet. Yet the doctor seemed so sure that the patch was in its place and the elevation changes should not impact anything. My advice to others, be your own advocate, if something doesn't make sense or your instincts say your not fully healed give yourself more time.

Some additional information in all of this that is important for the reader is my ear issue at this time was not my only health challenge. It was just before this visit that I found out some other health challenges that I had to face that created the need to step down from my position as a Branch Manager. It was this day where I felt like ok, what else can happen? Over the months following this appointment I had up and down days, trying to see something positive in the hole in the ear.

After seeing the ENT last spring and finding out that I would indeed need a hearing aid, I can recall not being ready to believe it. Even when people would ask me why I am I talking too loud...or when I would have to say what or be trying to focus so hard to hear something, I did not want to believe it. I also knew that I could not afford to purchase a hearing aid. The cost of them is something one has to plan for in most cases. It's like the purchase of an expensive computer or a cheap car depending on how you want to look at it.

Someone who has a hearing loss has to be mentally ready, financially ready, and physically ready before they can take the step towards purchasing a hearing aid even when it is something they need. It is not just as simple as some may think.

Over the spring and summer of 2018, I spent many days not fully being able to hear. At work customers at times would say something and I would have to ask them to repeat it and still not get what they said fully. Yet I would hear a noise, it is like I can hear there is something going on but can not hear the words. Like I am talking through glass all of the time or someone is talking to me through a wall. With that being said, certain people who have louder voices sometimes I can hear them where others I can not. Those who have higher pitched voices I struggle with the most. I can recall going to several choir concerts for my kids Spring and Winter 2018 and being able to hear the music but not the words.

It was through this time of not being able to hear and recognizing that hearing was not coming back that I mentally prepared for the need of my hearing aid. Something important to note for those in the life of someone getting a hearing aid, they probably are not ready for it when they actually get the hearing aid. They are just coming to grips with the reality of the situation and are trying the best they can to be prepared for it.

Chapter 6

Breaking point

It was in the month of November 2018 where I realized I was coming to a breaking point with hearing in certain situations. Work had become extremely difficult to manage. I was leaving work feeling exhausted from the day. Not to say there had not been exhaustion before, but that it was breaking me down further each day where I found it hard to get out of bed the next day, or to have a conversation with anyone. I almost did not want to talk to anyone.

The act of having a conversation when you have hearing loss can be a process especially if not in a quiet room, background noise makes a huge impact. To those reading this book that may have someone in their life who has a hearing loss, my suggestion would be to be patient. A person may seem withdrawn on some level if they do not talk as much as they did prior to the hearing loss. They may also at times talk to loud, or too quiet and it will likely not be at the right time or place. This in itself was a part of the breaking point of knowing it was time to purchase a hearing aid.

Chapter 7

Hearing aid Purchase

When one is mentally prepared as much as they can be to purchase their hearing aid they should also be financially prepared. I can say I was not ready financially for this. A recommendation that I would have to all people, including those that are healthy is to have a plan for health problems. A nest egg set aside just for the purpose of paying for medical expenses. If someone ever asked me if I would have medical problems that would include the hearing loss at my age, I would never have believed them. I was lucky to have a few small donations towards my hearing aid along with a bigger gift from my boyfriend to help get me to the goal of purchasing the hearing aid.

The first step in purchasing a hearing aid is to decide the best price, brand, and features that you want. One of the most important items for me was the cost. Most places sell a hearing aid for over $2000 per hearing aid. However, Costco sells them at wholesale so this is a good place to purchase for the value. With that being said in the following sections of this book read more as to reconsider purchasing from Costco if money is not an issue.

The second important feature to me was control over the hearing aid functions. Some hearing aids have the ability to use an app on your cell phone to change features depending on one's environment. For some size might be an importance, but it was not at the top of the list. It did not matter if it was big and bulky as long as I could hear, and people didn't have to hear me talk loud. I have become sensitive to this as I feel bad that sometimes I just can not tell how loud I am talking.

A recommendation that I have for those buying a hearing aid is to be your own advocate. When I was purchasing the hearing aid one of the employees at costco was trying to steer me in a direction, even though I had already performed my own research and clearly stated what I wanted. I knew I wanted a hearing aid I could control based on my surroundings. Example of this is if I go to a music concert I want to be able to hear the words and may need to adjust features to make that work. As I am not a hearing aid expert I suggest one to perform their own research, but I found I preferred the Resound hearing aid that I could connect to my smart-phone and adjust.

After wearing hearing aids for the first time I noticed a profound difference. I recall crying happy tears when I realized the difference it actually makes in my life. How I did not have to say "what" as often, how I could hear words at a concert and not just the music, how I could talk to someone without them thinking I am yelling. I can recall people at work and in my personal life asking me why I was talking so loud all of the time. When you have a hearing loss it is a challenge to know how loud you are talking, which can be a problem in many scenarios. Consider working in a small space and talking with clients about confidential information, yet everyone in the building can hear you. Don't wait, if you think or have been told would benefit from a hearing aid.

Chapter 8

Challenges

Some challenges I have faced since getting hearing aid is that after wearing all day the back of my ear hurts. I believe this stems from the surgical incision still being tender nearly two years after the Meatoplasty surgery. When the environment changes, sometimes it takes a moment to regulate the change and adjust to the change in volume when speaking. A second challenge that I face is pain on the inside of the ear, not related to the hearing aid but likely due to the patch partially being obstructed or to pressure changes. When answers are not clear it can prove frustrating, but I have found trying to remain positive that today is a rough day but tomorrow it will be better helps me.

Further loss of hearing has happened in the 9 months since getting hearing aid. I have noticed that I have to raise the volume of the hearing aid. Part of me was prepared for this based on a conversation had with the ENT that part of the patch had come off and repeating the surgery would likely result in similar results. The patch will likely have a challenge staying in place due the pressure in my ears.

Focusing on why does something like this happen does not help solve the problem. So I try to remain positive, do the best I can to hear what I can and not talk loud and I prepare for the future. In the coming years I will have to get a hearing aid for my right ear to help compensate for the hearing loss in both ears. Preparing and planning for this event will help when the time comes.

Chapter 9

Important considerations

A few things to keep in mind when talking to someone with a hearing impairment. Try not to put people on speaker phone when you are talking to them. Hearing through speaker has significant background noise and in many cases the person will not be able to hear you clearly. Be patient, sometimes the person will not hear you and they will say "what" more than you may like. It could be the environment, or it could be any number of things. Keep in mind that the person was paying attention, but if there is a lot going on it may be a struggle to focus and hear an entire conversation. Minimize playing music when your having a conversation as this puts extra listening challenges on the person. Recognize that a person may opt to not go out somewhere if it is a loud environment, and be flexible to going somewhere quiet such that you can have a conversation that both parties or a group can be a part of. And finally looking at the person when speaking as it directs the best volume towards the person.

Final thoughts

As I close out this first version of 'A whole in the ear' I want to thank those in my life who have been patient through the process. And give advice to those who may be struggling with a similar problem, maybe it is hearing loss, or maybe another health challenge. Remember that while it may seem challenging today, you will get through this and believe it or not, will learn something about yourself that you didn't know. Something I learned, I am stronger than I ever gave myself credit, and that I needed to work on being a better listener. Find what you can learn from your experience, focus on how you can grow, and be your own advocate.